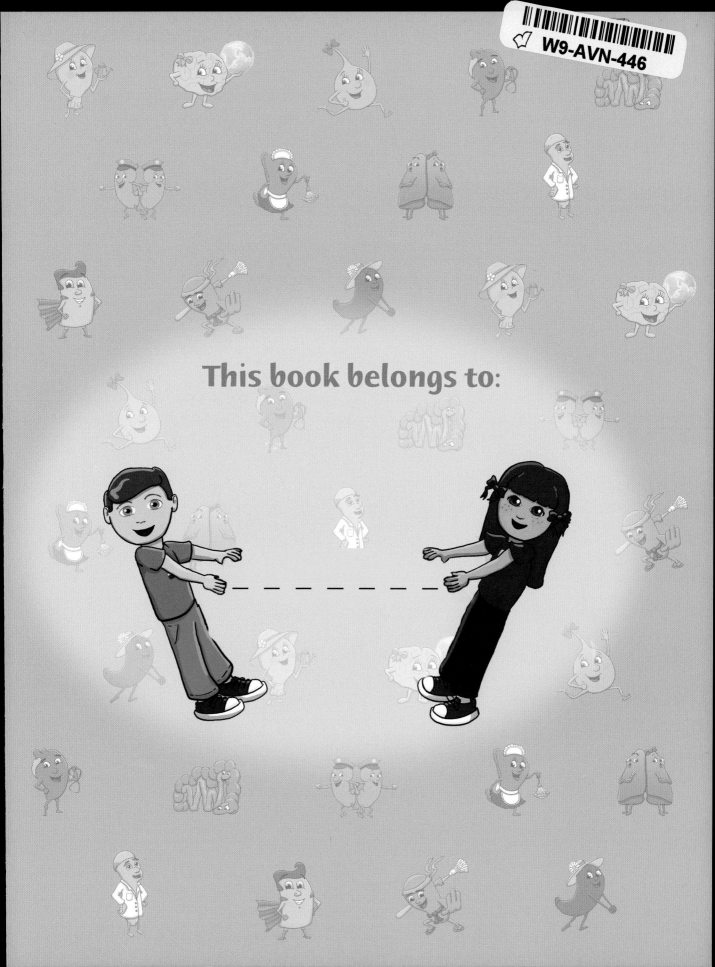

This book belongs to:

I would like to dedicate this book to my wonderful grandchildren:
Mikayla and Matthew. May *Ana-Tommy and Friends* help you see
the importance of taking care of your amazing bodies.

And . . .

To children everywhere: our hope for the future.

Lina Anton-Echeverria

This book was created with help from a number of remarkable
people that worked together as a team.

Thanks to Chevy, for believing in my idea and supporting
and helping me to keep the project moving forward.

Thanks to Aaron, who through his musical talent gave me
the inspiration to start this project.

Thanks to Veronica, Kellee, and Natasha for their help
in completing this project.

Ana-Tommy, Inc., San Diego, CA 92101
Copyright © 2012 Ana-Tommy and Friends, Making Anatomy Fun!
www.ana-tommy.com

The intent of the author is only to offer information of a general nature. If you have questions regarding
how the information applies to your child, speak to your child's health-care provider.
The author and publisher assume no responsibility for misuse of the information provided.

Printed in the United States of America by Worzalla, July 2012
ISBN-978-0-9840079-0-5 First Edition
Library of Congress Control Number 2012910809
Ana-Tommy and Friends, Making Anatomy Fun!/Lina Anton-Echeverria

Ana-Tommy and Friends

Making Anatomy Fun!

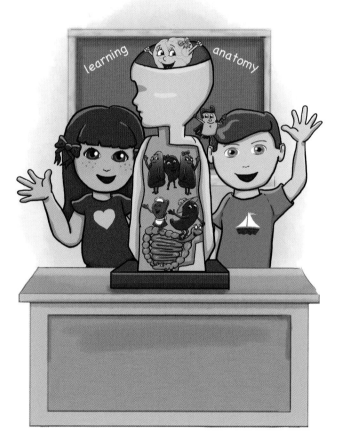

By Lina Anton-Echeverria

Characters created by Bianca Echeverria
Rhymes by Amber Plaster

A Note from the Author

The idea for *Ana-Tommy and Friends* came about from my concern with the increase of health problems among young people in today's society, and from my desire to do something to help.

Most importantly, my purpose is to help give children the knowledge to understand and appreciate their bodies and the motivation to make healthy choices.

Realizing my purpose turned out to be the easy part. Figuring out how to share what I'd learned in a fun and impactful way was more difficult. There are many books that explain what the organs are and how they function. I wanted to create something different from what already existed. My goal is to bring information to life, so that children could bridge the gap between memorizing facts and actually understanding why they need to care for their bodies.

Most children can't name their organs, don't understand how they work, and aren't able to visualize the inside of their bodies. I want kids to be able to visualize where their livers are, in the same way that they can picture where their noses are. Allowing those dreams to guide me, I created *Ana-Tommy and Friends*.

Creating *Ana-Tommy and Friends* has truly been a labor of love. My heart is full when I see children and parents light up with excitement as they make the connection between what the characters are describing and what is happening inside their own bodies. It is truly my hope that *Ana-Tommy and Friends* will help children learn to value all that is within them, body and soul.

Lina Anton-Echeverria

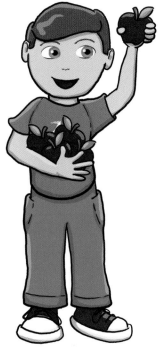

A Note to Parents

The beauty of *Ana-Tommy and Friends* is that there is something here for children of all ages. Children love the sound of rhyming verses.

Take notice as you read each rhyme to your child for the first couple of times. By the third or fourth time you read *Ana-Tommy and Friends* to your child, pause before saying the second line of the rhyme. You might be surprised to find that your child may supply the next verse for you, depending on the child's pace of learning. This will show you that your child is paying attention to rhyming sounds.

Two very important teaching tools when reading are patience and the desire to share your own love of reading.

Enjoy your reading experience!

Lina Anton-Echeverria

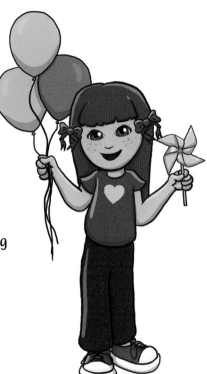

Ana

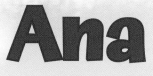

My name is Ana.
I'm a kid just like you.
I have some new friends
that you should know too.

They are called "organs,"
and as you will see,
if I care for them,
they will care for me.

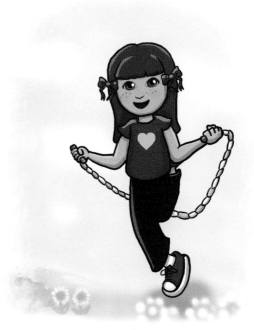

They live in a wonderful place. Can you guess where?
Inside our bodies! Did you know they were there?

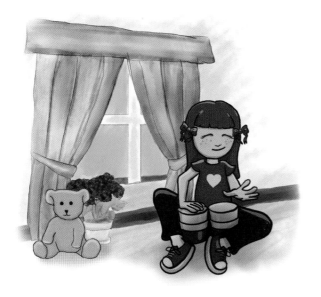

But first let's meet Tommy.
He's a good friend of mine.
Then we'll all learn together,
and have a good time!

Tommy

I'm Ana's friend Tommy,
and I'm learning with you
that organs are living
in my body too!

We have the same organs,
just like you.
A heart, brain, and stomach,
to name just a few.

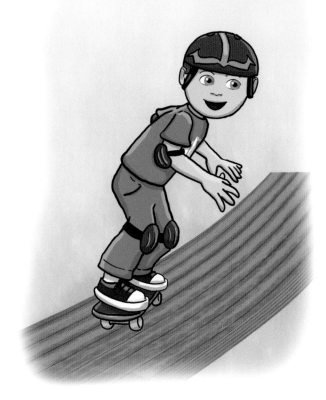

I have many questions. There's a lot I don't know.
What are their jobs? Will they help me to grow?

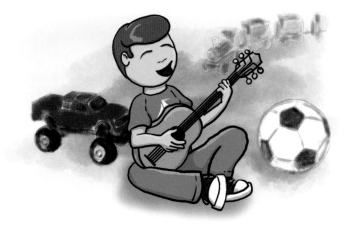

Let's start off by meeting
Brianna the Brain.
She's always in charge,
so we'll let her explain.

Brianna the Brain

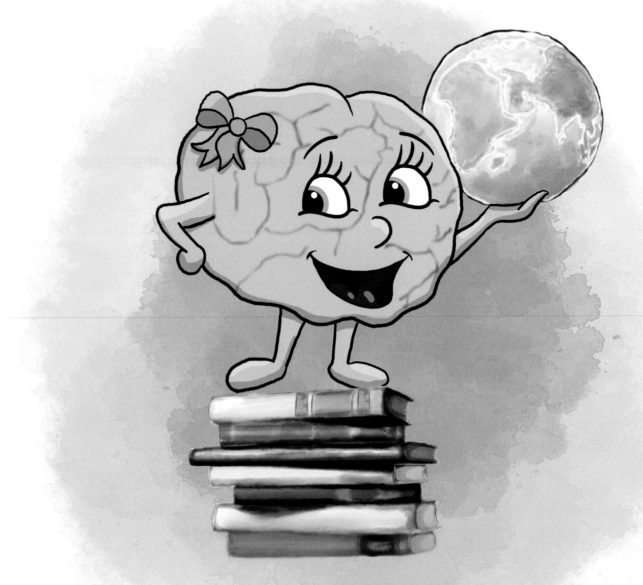

My name is Brianna, Brianna the Brain.
I help you remember your age and your name.
One of my jobs is to help you grow,
not too fast, and not too slow.

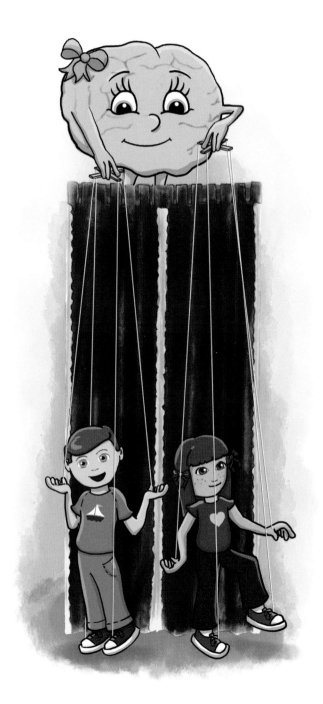

Do you wonder how you
breathe, blink, or think?
It's me! I keep your whole
body in sync.

I talk to your lungs,
your eyes, and your heart,
to all of your muscles
and all of your parts.

I hold dreams and memories
and help you retain
all that you learn.
I'm Brianna the Brain.

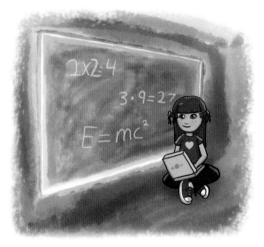

Dart the Heart

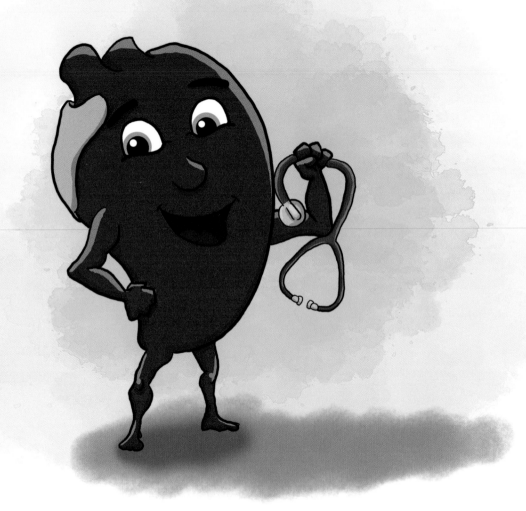

I'm Dart the Heart. Guess what I do?
I move your blood inside of you!
I push it through tubes called "arteries" and "veins,"
down to your toes and up to your brain.

I'm a strong muscle inside your chest.
I work night and day, never stopping to rest.
I beat slowly when you sleep and fast when you run.
I'm Dart the Heart, getting things done.

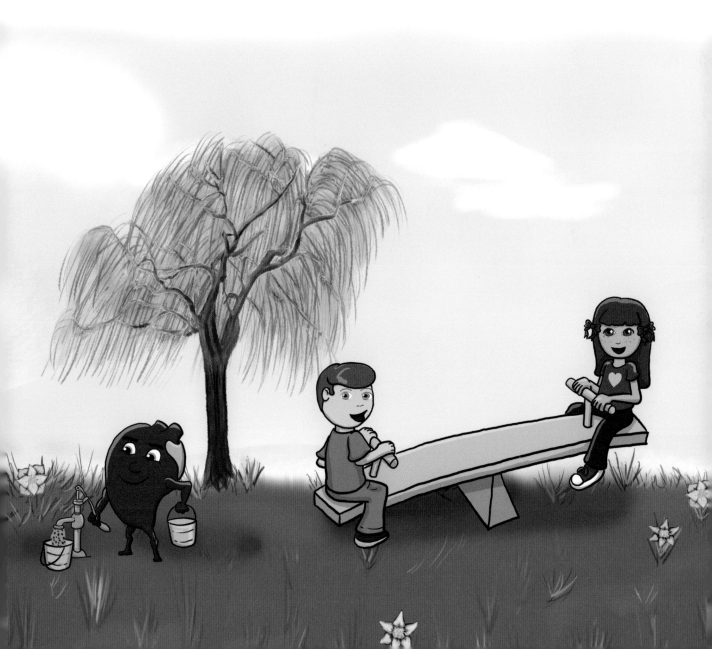

Leo and Lea the Lungs

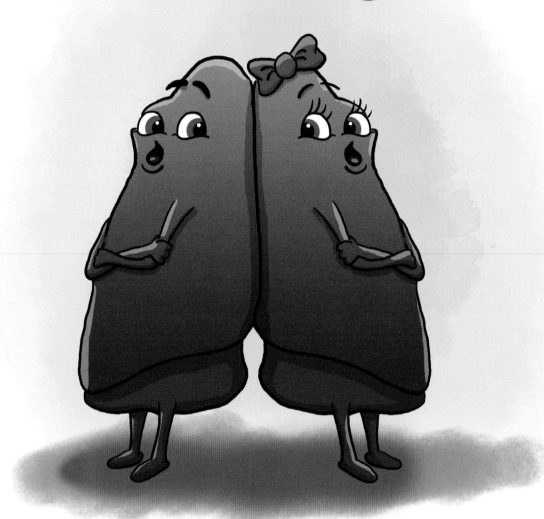

We are Leo and Lea, we work as a pair.
We are your lungs, and we help you breathe air.
Protected by ribs, sitting safe in your chest,
we do more than breathe. Have you already guessed?

When you sing or laugh,
talk or shout,
we are the ones
helping you out.

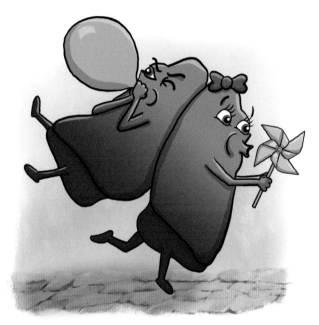

Take a deep breath.
Feel the rise in your chest.
Let it all out; take a spilt-second rest.
Inhaling and exhaling is a job
we both share.
We are Leo and Lea,
the breathing pair.

Tammy the Tummy

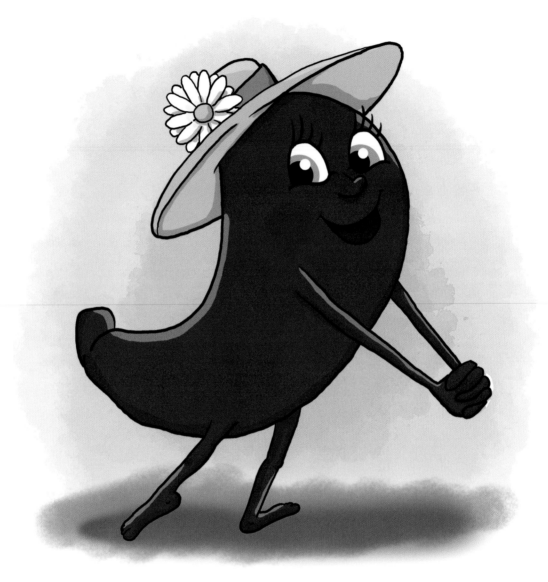

I am Tammy, your little tummy.
I store the food you thought was yummy.
I mix it up, and I break it down.
Sometimes I make a funny sound.

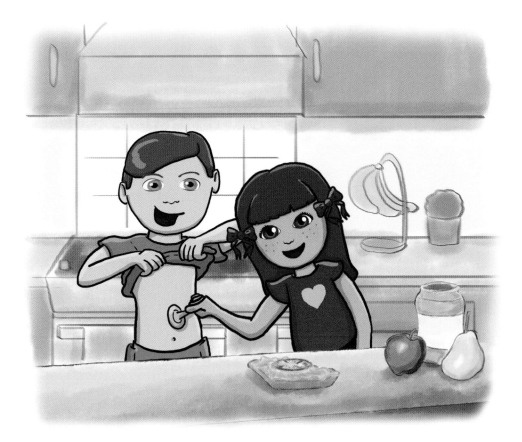

When I am hungry, I'll let you know.
You'll feel a grumble down below.
Whatever it is you like to eat,
be sure to make your meals complete.

Give me food that isn't crummy,
and I'll help you feel good.
I'm Tammy the Tummy.

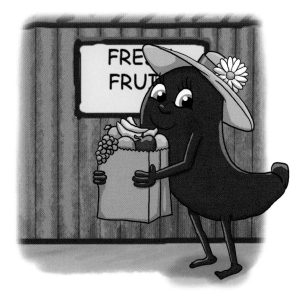

Lily the Liver

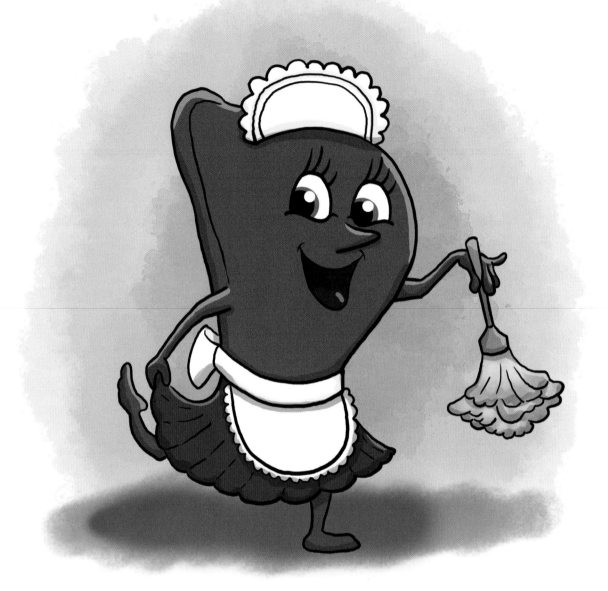

I am Lily, Lily the Liver.
All of your clean blood is what I deliver.
I make a fluid called "bile" that breaks down fat
and helps with digestion. How amazing is that?

I absorb the vitamins
that your body needs,
and also help heal a cut
when it bleeds.

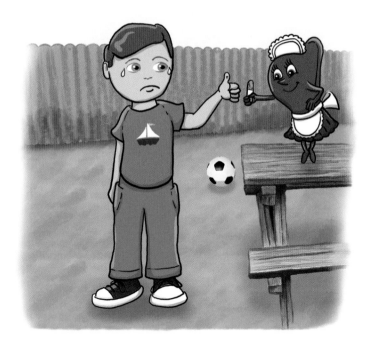

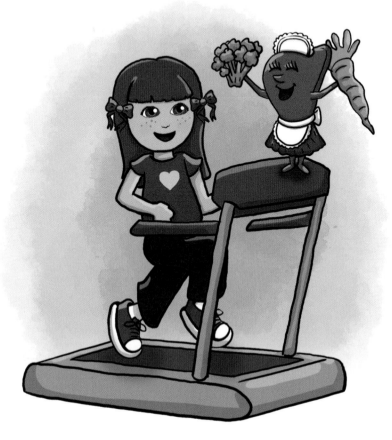

I'm a serious worker
with no time to be silly.
I sit right in your belly.
I'm the Liver named Lily.

Gail the Gallbladder

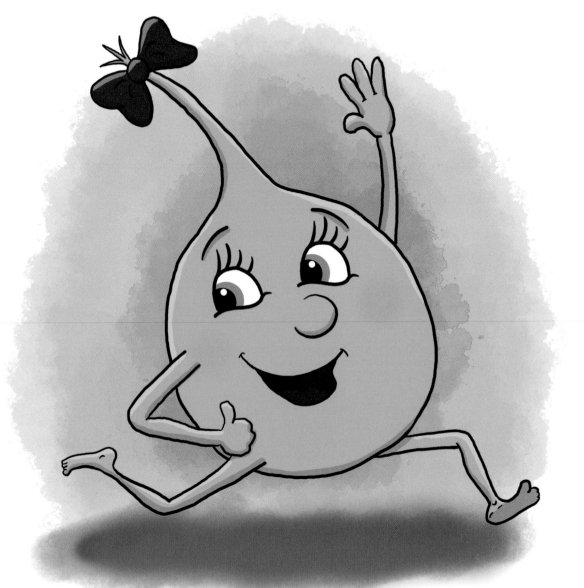

I'm the little gallbladder. My name is Gail.
Think of me as Lily's trash pail.
When Lily is finished making her bile,
she gives it to me to hold for a while.

I keep the bile from becoming dense,
by holding in the water. Does that make more sense?

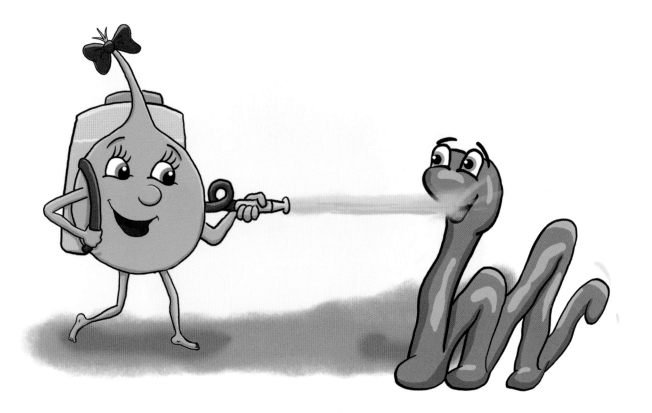

I squeeze out the bile to help with digestion,
as your food makes its way to the small intestine.
I'm just another part of the "digestive trail."
I'm the little gallbladder, and my name is Gail.

Pete the Pancreas

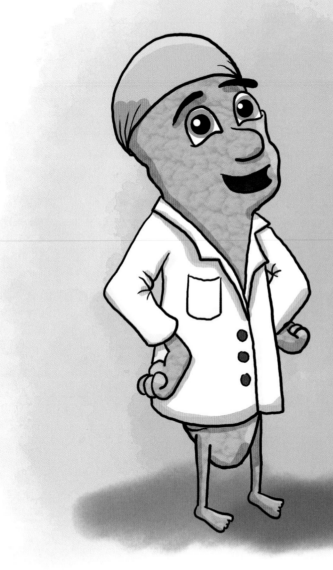

I'm your Pancreas.
My name is Pete.
I'm an organ and a gland.
Wow! Isn't that neat?

I'm long and flat, and rather little.
Touch your stomach and your back —
I'm there in the middle!
I help neutralize acids, but not only that.
I also break down carbs, protein, and fat.
In addition, I store sugar away,
in case you may need it another day.
I release hormones
every time that you eat.
I am your pancreas.
My name is Pete.

Weston and Preston the Intestines

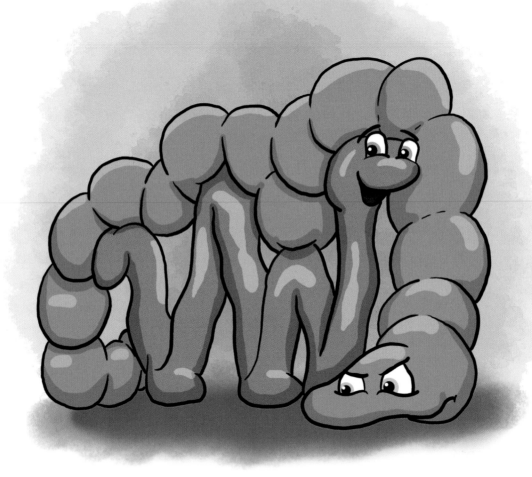

We are Weston and Preston,
the small and large intestines.
We are the last place
your food will digest in.

Some people call us
"guts" as well.
In your belly is
where we dwell.

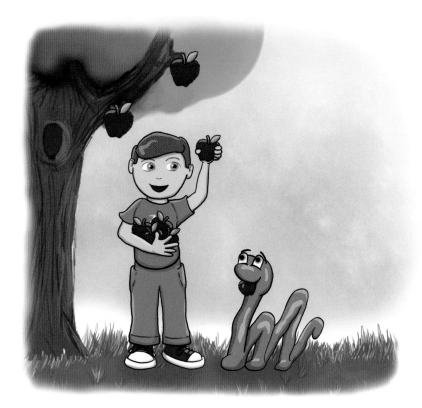

Once in a while, Preston will pass
some little bubbles.
Did you know it was gas?
We pull the last bits of nutrients out
before sending your "poop" to its exiting route.

We finish the job, that's what
we are best in.
We're Weston and Preston,
your team of intestines.

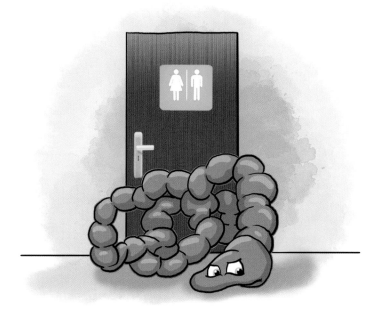

Sonny the Spleen

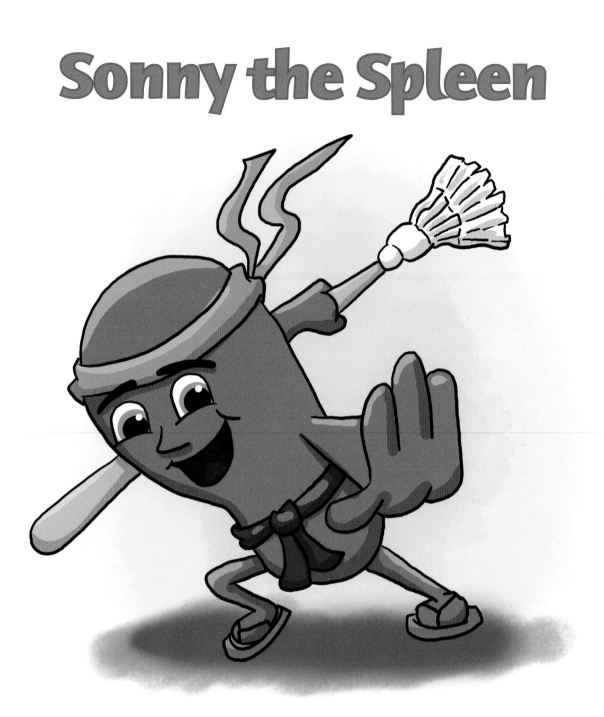

Hey there kids! I'm Sonny the Spleen.
Fighting germs is my daily routine.
I watch out for those little offenders,
because I'm a warrior, a fighter, your body's defender!

I may be small, weighing less than a pound,
but I remove bad bacteria wherever it's found.
I break down old cells
that your blood needs to lose,
and recycle iron for new cells to use.
I'm known as a tissue-healing machine
that fights infections. I'm Sonny the Spleen.

Kyle and Kimmy the Kidneys

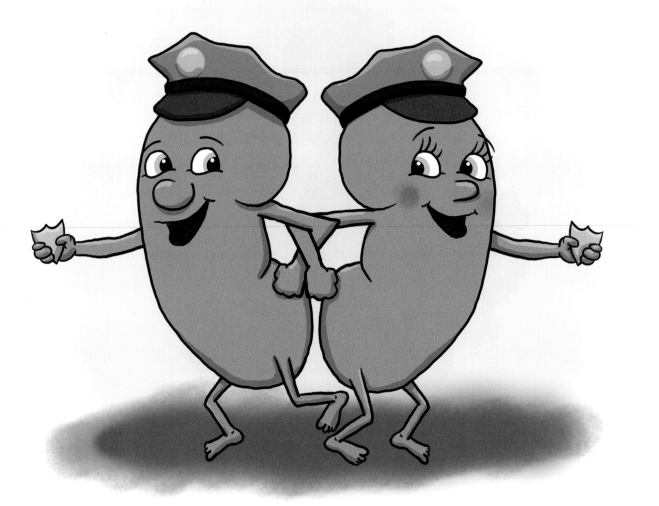

We are Kyle and Kimmy,
the cool kidney pack.
We are shaped like beans
in the middle of your back.

We filter your blood,
and as it goes through,
we take out the waste
and dispose it for you.
We mix waste with water
that turns into "pee"
and balance your body's chemistry!
When it comes to waste,
we do not slack.
We are Kyle and Kimmy,
the cool kidney pack.

Bailey the Bladder

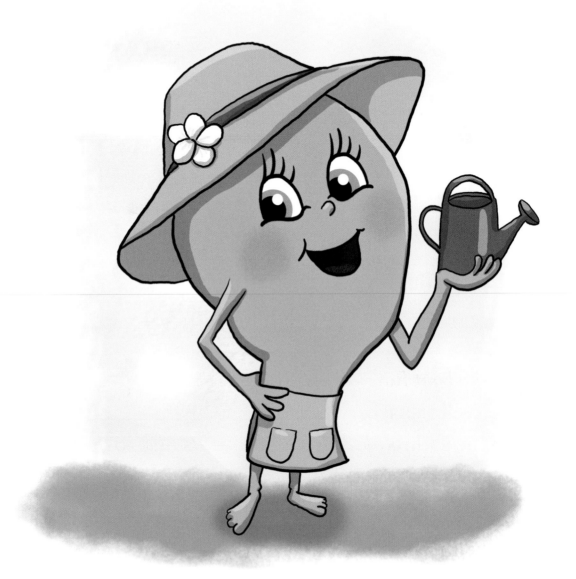

I'm Bailey the Bladder.

How I help is no small matter.

You can think of me like a small tank.

I hold all of the liquids that you drank.

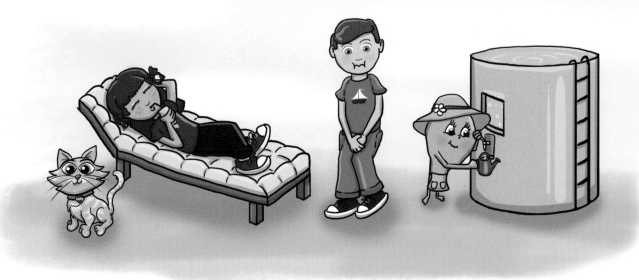

When I get full, I let Brianna know.
She will signal back, "It's time to go!"
To the bathroom, that is, because it's time to get free,
from the build up of the yellowish liquid you call "pee!"
After I empty, your belly will feel flatter,
until I fill up again! I'm Bailey the Bladder.

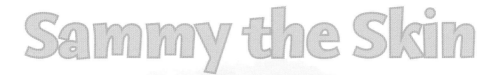

Sammy the Skin

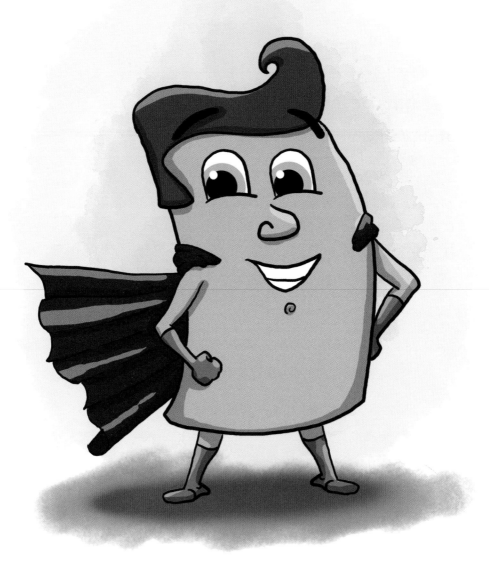

I am Sammy the Skin. Guess what I do?
I protect all the organs inside of you!
I come in shades from dark to light,
no matter your color, it is just right.

I help you feel
all the things that you hold,
soft and hard, hot and cold.
I keep your body
temperature right,
during a hot day or a very cold night.

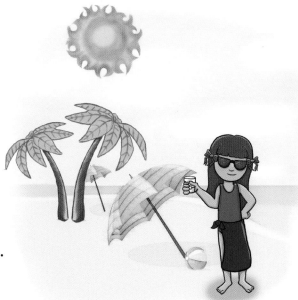

I replace dead skin cells and heal a wound from within.
I'm stretchy and strong. I'm Sammy the Skin.

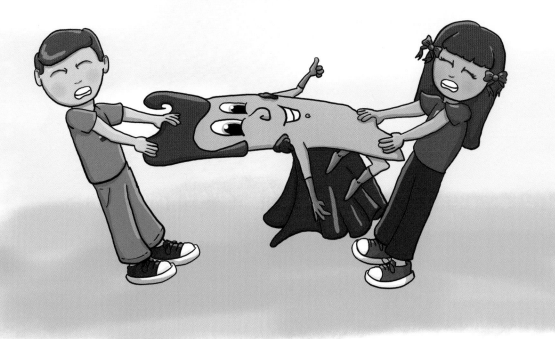

Now that you've met some of our friends,
just remember this is not where it ends.
We have many exciting adventures in store.
Join us next time, and you'll learn so much more.
Exercise! Eat healthy! Show your body you care,
and always remember to read, learn, and share.

Glossary

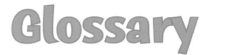

Absorb To take something in.

Acids Body fluids with a sour or bitter taste.

Arteries Vessels that carry blood from your heart to the rest of your body.

Bacteria An organism that is usually single celled and may contain helpful or harmful material.

Bile A yellow-green liquid made by the liver. It is stored in the gallbladder and helps you digest your food.

Carbs A group of organic compounds (including sugars, starches, celluloses, and gums) that serves as a major energy source.

Cells Small functional units that make up tissue and organisms.

Chemistry How substances react to each other.

Concentrate To make (a solution or mixture) less dilute.

Defender To protect from harm.

Dense Thick, crowded closely together.

Digest To break down food so that it can be absorbed into the bloodstream and used by the body.

Digestion The process of breaking down food and separating from it the things that the body needs.

Digestive	The process of breaking down food.
Dispose	To get rid of something.
Dwell	To live in a place.
Exiting	The act of going out, or leaving.
Fat	An oily substance found in the body tissue.
Filter	A device that cleans liquids as they pass through.
Gland	An organ in the body that produces or releases natural chemicals.
Healing	A process by which the body repairs itself.
Hormones	Substances produced by a tissue that helps your body function.
Infections	An illness caused by Infections can be viral or bacterial in nature and might be caused by a fungus or parasite.
Iron	A mineral essential for life, present in every living cell.
Neutralize	Of or relating to a solution or compound that is neither acidic nor alkaline.
Nutrients	A substance, such as protein, a mineral, or a vitamin, that is needed by people, animals, and plants to stay strong and healthy.

Offenders	Something that offends and causes displeasure.
Organ	Parts of the body, such as the heart or kidneys, that have a certain purpose.
Protein	A type of chemical compound in all living things.
Recycle	To reuse.
Retain	To keep in mind.
Route	A path of travel.
Routine	A regular sequence of actions.
Sync	If things are in sync, they work well together.
Tissue	A mass of similar cells that form a particular part of an organ.
Veins	Vessels through which blood is sent back to the heart from other parts of the body.
Vitamins	Substances in food that are essential for good health and nutrition.
Warrior	Someone who fights with courage and determination.
Waste	What the body does not use or need after it is done digesting.

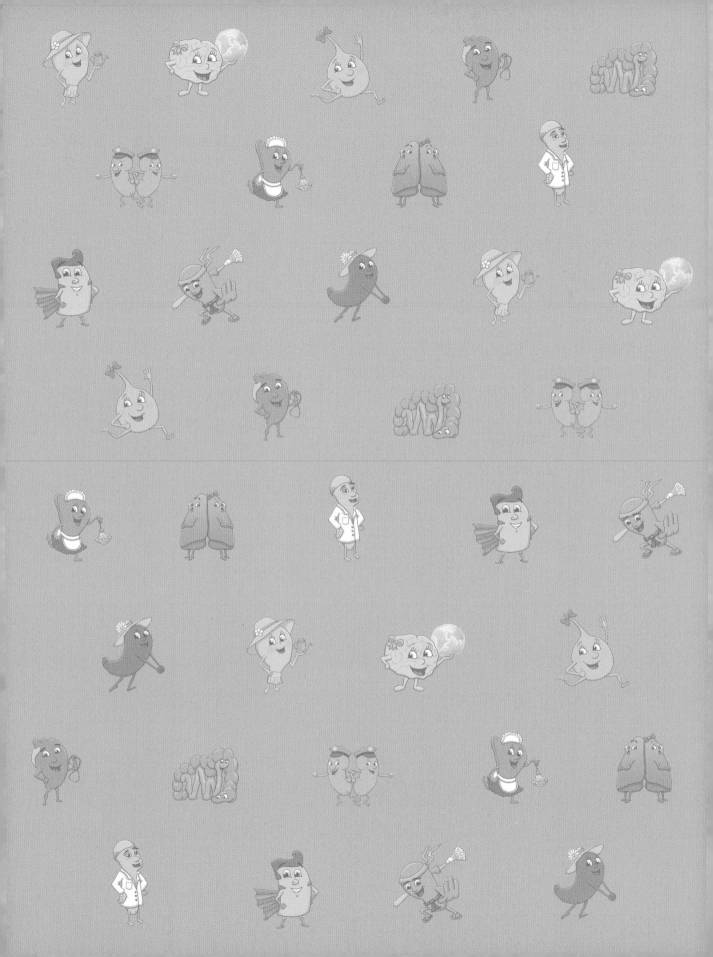